Intermittent Fasting For Women

An Improved Beginner's Guide to Fast Weight Loss and Effective Fat Burn

By Belinda Watts

Disclaimer

The content in this book is not intended to diagnose or treat any disease or condition, nor function as a substitute for medical advice. Please consult your physician before beginning any treatment for an existing medical condition. You must not rely on the information in this book as an alternative to medical advice from your doctor or other professional healthcare provider. You should never delay seeking medical treatment nor disregard medical advice because of the information in this book.

The publisher and author of this book shall not be held liable or responsible for any misunderstanding or misuse of the content contained in this book or for any loss, damage, or injury caused or alleged to be caused directly or indirectly be any treatment, action, or application of any information discussed in this book.

Copyright © 2016 Belinda Watts

All rights reserved. No part of this publication may be reproduced, stored in a retrieval system, or transmitted, in any form or by any means, electronic, mechanical, photocopying, recording or otherwise, without prior written permission of the owner, except for inclusion of brief quotations in a review.

Table of Contents

Introduction

Chapter 1: What is Intermittent Fasting?

Chapter 2: How Does Intermittent Fasting Work?

Chapter 3: Benefits of Intermittent Fasting

Chapter 4: Common Myths of Intermittent Fasting

Chapter 5: Popular Fasting Methods and Programs

Chapter 6: Proof that Intermittent Fasting Works

Conclusion

Introduction

Hello, Ladies! I want to thank you and congratulate you for downloading *Intermittent Fasting For Women: An Improved Beginner's Guide to Fast Weight Loss and Effective Fat Burn!* We all know the struggle of losing weight, it's not an easy journey by any means. And with dozens of different programs all guaranteeing you a "bikini ready body," just choosing a weight loss method becomes a challenge of its own. Of course you want to pick a plan that gives you the most drastic results in the shortest amount of time; but it is almost impossible to lose a significant amount of weight in just a few weeks.

Many weight loss programs center around incorporating a vigorous exercise program that has the stamp of approval from a handful of professionals. But the truth is that you don't need exercise in order to completely transform your body, although it does help. Many of us have jobs, family, and other obligations that keep us from hitting the gym; just the thought of spending an hour doing something for yourself can seem unrealistic. But your body composition is mostly influenced by what you eat. Being fit or looking leaner is 80 percent diet and just 20 percent of exercise. Although I am not discounting the many benefits and effects of exercising, I am saying that as long as you focus on building good eating habits, you will experience amazing results!

Although eating right is crucial for building a strong foundation for weight loss success, the greatest thing you can do for your body is fast. Fasting is when you only consume water for a predetermined amount of time in order to experience incredible health benefits. In hardly any time at all, you will see amazing results. A complete fast is typically twenty-one days long. However, with so much going on in your life, it can be challenging to commit so much effort towards such a strenuous task. That is why intermittent fasting is the best option for you!

Intermittent fasting allows you to enjoy the foods you love while still losing weight and experiencing all of the other many benefits fasting has to offer. Intermittent fasting is simple and can be done by anyone who has the self-discipline to improve their mind, body, and soul. This book contains proven steps and strategies on how to become a true expert of intermittent fasting for the female body. Because, let's face it, every weight loss program is not really a "one size fits all" method of weight loss.

Here is an inescapable fact: men and women lose weight differently. Our bodies are not the same, and therefore are effect differently according to our diet and exercise regiments. Just like with any other weight loss program, if you fast incorrectly, you could experience harmful or concerning effects or conditions that may inhibit the proper function of your body's systems. If you do not develop your knowledge and technique of intermittent fasting, then you may end up putting your body in danger. This book will explain what intermittent fasting is, its benefits and side- effects, how to properly implement fasting into your daily life, and much, much more!

It's time for you to become a better and healthier you! Self-improvement begins with one small step that influences you to alter your lifestyle. Reading this book is your first step to becoming a whole new you! Just remember that great changes come from continuous effort, self- motivation, and time. If you believe in yourself and the person that you aspire to become, then nothing can stop you from achieving your fitness and weight loss goals! Good luck on your journey of self- improvement and enjoy!

Chapter 1: What is Intermittent Fasting?

A Brief History of Fasting

Fasting is an ancient practice that has been around for hundreds of thousands of years! Many cultures and religions regularly practice fasting for its many medical benefits and spiritual guidance. The history of fasting does not have a known beginning because it is considered to be a normal part of the human existence. Even most animals will fast during times of illness or stress; as fasting brings rest, balance, and conserves your energy. Although many people today believe that fasting is another form of starvation or think that it should not be considered a common medical practice, philosophers and physicians of the past have agreed that fasting is an ancient fundamental process that is vital for curing sick organisms.

Hippocrates, Socrates, Galen, Plato, and Aristotle were a handful of philosophers who spoke about the physical and spiritual renewal that fasting could bring. Paracelsus, who is one of the three fathers of Wester medicine, believed that fasting is the greatest remedy to illness. Early medical practices regarded fasting as a method of revitalizing and rejuvenating the body.

Most early religions and spiritual organizations regularly implemented fasting as a part of rituals and ceremonies, typically during fall and spring equinoxes. Christianity, Buddhism, Judaism, Hinduism, Islam, and Gnosticism exercise multiple forms of fasting. Religious or spiritual fasting has been performed for purification, penance, sacrifice, spiritual vision, divine communication, and mourning. Roman Catholics and the Eastern Orthodox Church fast through the observation of Lent, which lasts for forty days. Judaism has multiple annual fasts, such as Yom Kippur. And in Islam, Muslims will fast during the sacred month of Ramadan. Although spiritual fasting began thousands of years ago, major religions continue practices of fasting even today for spiritual prosperity.

Fasting has also been found in Native American tribes, typically practiced before going to war and in coming-of-age rituals. It was even believed amongst Native Americans that fasting assuaged angry deities to avoid natural catastrophes, such as floods or famine.

In more recent times, fasting has been used as an expression of political protests. Women's rights suffragettes and Mahatma Gandhi are just two examples of hunger strike protests. There are also yoga practicing individuals who include fasting as part of their exercise for achieving meditation or spiritual intuition.

Intermittent Fasting vs. Absolute Fasting

Before we dive into different fasting methods and the benefits of fasting, it is important to understand the difference between intermittent fasting and absolute fasting. Intermittent fasting is a technique that allows you to experience the benefits of a full fast without straining your body and mind as much as a full fast would.

Fasting is when you willingly abstain from consuming food, drink, or both from a predetermined period of time. Fasting can also be limiting your intake of food so drastically that your body still enters the desired metabolic state. The fasting period typically lasts for twenty-four hours, however there are cases when an individual has fasted for twenty-one days and even forty days. The purpose of completing such a demanding task is to allow your body to completely detox and heal from toxins and other ailments that have inhibited your health. It takes a full twenty- one day fast for every cell in your body to regenerate new, healthy cells.

Water fasting is the most common form of fasting. During a water fast, you are only allowed to consume water during the fasting period. There are also juice fasts and meticulous calorie restricted fasts that allow you to consume only certain foods. All of these examples represent methods of absolute fasting.

Intermittent fasting is not as vigorous as absolute fasting. Intermittent fasting is fasting for a much shorter timeframe. Instead of fasting for a few days or weeks, you fast for a few hours at a time several times a week. Intermittent fasting, or IF, involves skipping one or more meals a day in order to lose weight. I know, skipping breakfast probably goes against everything your mom told you as a child. But many studies have shown that breakfast may not be as important as society has made it out to be. Skipping breakfast has actually been proven to help individuals lose weight. This also may sound contradictory to what many diet programs instruct you to do. Dr. Oz, Medi-Weightloss, and other plans lead you to believe that eating six small meals a day will help you lose weight. These plans are based on the theory that consuming multiple meals keeps your metabolism working at maximum capacity all day. While this method may work in theory, it leads dieters to eat more so that their metabolism is only burning what they just ate, rather than the fat cells that have already been stored.

The reality is your body does not need food every three or four hours. Habitual eating weighs down your digestive system, leads to over eating, and causes severe weight gain. Through intermittent fasting, you will be skipping breakfast and eating less during your meals so that you are in a caloric deficit; which in turn makes your body feed off of the fat that is has already stored. Intermittent fasting is not necessarily a diet, but a dieting pattern and lifestyle. You are purposely skipping a meal or two during your fasting period while still eating good food the rest of the time.

Intermittent fasting is when you only eat during a window of time during the day. Most IF participants will only eat between noon and eight at night, giving a solid eight hour period where they can consume one or two meals and a snack. Other fasters choose to perform a full twenty- four hour fast, skipping every meal for an entire day. For example: if your last meal was dinner at six o'clock at night, your next meal won't be until six o'clock the following night.

Intermittent fasting is typically performed every day, which is why it is considered a lifestyle, rather than a diet. Most people who do intermittent fasting will adapt it as a regular part of their life, rather than a temporary solution to weight loss or body cleansing. While it may sound intimidating to change your lifestyle as a long-term investment to better health, you actually already fast every single day! Yes, you are already a fasting expert without even knowing it! You fast every night when you are sleeping, which can be between six to eight hours of not eating. With intermittent fasting, all you are doing is prolonging when you eat "breakfast" in order to lose weight.

Up next you are going to learn the science behind intermittent fasting. Everyone knows that if you don't eat, you will lose weight. But how and why is this so? How does intermittent fasting work when you are still eating full meals every day? In the next chapter, I will break down how your body functions during an intermittent fast so you can understand the full process of fasting.

Chapter 2: How Does Intermittent Fasting Work?

Whenever you eat a meal, your body will use whatever food you just ate as energy. You have heard that carbohydrates are good for you because they give you energy, which is true in a sense. With the readily available sugar and starches that you have just consumed, it is easy for your body to burn them for energy in your blood stream. This means that your body will keep using the food you just ate for energy rather than the stored fat it already has.

When you eat a meal that has carbohydrates in it, you are consuming glucose, or sugar. When you consume glucose, your blood sugar levels rise. This causes the leptin in your body to release insulin from your pancreas. Leptin is a fat burning hormone, which makes it important when you are trying to lose weight. Eating too much sugar on a daily basis can give you type two diabetes, which means that your pancreas can no longer produce insulin. It can also lead to leptin resistance. Leptin resistance makes your body slow in responding to spikes in your blood sugar levels and leads to weight gain. When you consume too much sugar regularly, your leptin is constantly signaled. It is as if the glucose just stays in your bloodstream and soon your body begins to reflect the story *The Boy Who Cried Wolf*. Because your brain is constantly getting the signal to send leptin, it stops responding to your body's calls for it. You brain stops producing leptin and you begin to gain more weight.

Having high blood sugar levels is extremely dangerous, even deadly. Nearly every part of your body can be damaged by consuming too much blood sugar. The following is a list of the possible outcomes of eating and drinking too much sugar:

- Obesity

- Kidney disease

- Kidney failure

- Heart disease

- Heart attacks

- Strokes

- Erectile Dysfunction

- Vision loss

- Slow healing wounds

- A weakened immune system

- Nerve damage

- Poor circulation in the legs and feet

- Potential amputation

Any glucose that is not converted into energy for immediate use is then turned into glycogen and stored as fat. This is why too much sugary food leads to weight gain. Cutting down the amount of food and sugar you consume leads your body to use the excess fat cells for energy.

Your Body in a Fasting State

When you are in a fasting state, your body can no longer use food as a way to produce every, as you have not eaten anything. So then it is more likely to use the fat is has stored for energy. When you are fasting, your body produces its own energy by burning off excess carbohydrates and fats. Your liver is the most important organ during this process; the liver concerts fat cells into chemicals known as ketone bodies. Ketones are three water-soluble compounds, acetone, acetoacetic acid, and beta- hydroxybutyric acid, which are used for energy.

The state in which your body produces ketones to burn for energy is known as ketosis. During ketosis, your body burns pure fat cells, shrinking the size of your gut, thighs, and wherever else fat was stored. Ketones are produced when your body breaks down fats, which creates fatty acids that are burned off in the liver. This process is called beta-oxidation. This is why many people eat low carb, high fat diets; because it speeds up the process of getting your body into ketosis.

Ketosis is the ideal state that you want to enter when intermittent fasting, however, high levels of ketones are toxic. This condition is called ketoacidosis. When there is not enough insulin in your body, the condition can turn deadly. This is a condition similar to those with type one diabetes; if an individual who suffers from type one diabetes doesn't take insulin, especially during times of stress or illness, they can fall sick. Although this may make you wary of trying intermittent fasting, remember that you will not produce enough ketones during your fasting state to develop ketoacidosis. You will begin eating in just a few hours, which will ideally knock you out of a ketogenic state.

While going through the feast period of intermittent fasting, it is important to eat enough protein, fats, and carbs so your liver functions properly. Protein is converted into glucose when consumed, which is why eating too much of it can cause your body to stop ketosis. And the right amount of good fats will help you lose weight. Have a balanced feasting period is important because if you do not eat enough protein, your body will burn your muscle tissue to make the glucose it needs to thrive.

Intermittent fasting teaches your body to use the food it consumes more efficiently than it would with normal eating habits. When you fast, you are helping your body to use different nutrients for energy than the sugar it is used to relying on. When you fast, more growth hormone is released. This combined with the decrease in your insulin levels will result in muscle growth with fat loss. Not only will you become leaner through intermittent fasting, but you will become toned as well if you lift weights and go to the gym.

But weight loss and muscle growth are only two of the amazing benefits that intermittent fasting has to offer. In the next chapter, you will learn about the other great effects fasting has on your body and why so many people are implementing fasting as a part of their daily lives.

How Women React to Intermittent Fasting

Many women struggle with intense food cravings, especially during the time of their menstrual cycle. There are women who have tried intermittent fasting several times and failed miserably because of the violent roller coaster of cravings and heightened levels of energy followed by extreme lulls in energy. But accounts that are similar have been found with practically every diet out there for women who want to lose weight and create a healthy lifestyle. But while fad diets don't follow through with the promised results, intermittent fasting is highly effective for dedicated participants. The reality is that women experience intermittent fasting differently than men do. Although women can still experience the physiological and weight loss benefits of intermittent fasting, some ladies may need to take a different approach.

Women tend to react differently to intermittent fasting because of their hormones. IF can cause women to experience a hormonal imbalance, which can send mixed signals to their brains when fasting. Females are much more sensitive to signals of starvation. When the body senses starvation signals, it will increase the production of hunger hormones, which causes intense cravings for food. This can make breaking a fast more difficult; because when you begin eating after the fasting period, you will feel persistent hunger which can cause you to overeat. This natural reaction is your body's way of protecting an unborn baby, even if you are not actually pregnant. Even women with dedicated willpower fail during fasts and light meals and end up bingeing.

Sudden dramatic changes in eating habits can cause a lot of stress on your body and make your hormones go haywire. Once you have finished bingeing, it is suddenly time to start your fast again. Or maybe you realize the following day that you should cut your meals into smaller portions and end up eating less. The constant roller coaster of overeating followed by starvation can stop your ovulation. In some animal studies, it was shown that drastic intermittent fasting caused female lab rats to stop having menstrual cycles and their ovaries shrunk. Insomnia was another symptom that was found among some of the female rats.

There have been very few medical studies that have focused on the effects of intermittent fasting for women. But from what has been concluded in various lab animal studies has shown that intermittent fasting can sometimes change a woman's hormonal balance and lead to fertility issues. Here is a short list of symptoms that may indicate that you have a hormonal imbalance due to intermittent fasting:

- A bad or depressed mood

- Irregular periods

- Fatigue

- Headaches

- Bloating

However, if you listen to your body's signals and fully understand how to properly fast, then there is no reason why you should not experience all of the incredible benefits fasting has to offer. Because fasting is a lifestyle that you have to adapt to over a short period of time, it is important to realize when it is time for you to end a fast early or change your meals during the feasting period. The most effective way for you to ease your body into intermittent fasting is to start with shorter fasting periods; then over time, increase your fasting period until you can completely a full intermittent fast. As long as you are gentle on your body during fasting and eat wisely during your meals and are health conscience, then intermittent fasting will not negatively affect your health.

Chapter 3: Benefits of Intermittent Fasting

As you now know, fasting has been used for centuries as a cure for medical and spiritual healing. Fasting helps your body heal itself through cleansing out toxins and reproducing new and healthy cells that help your body function more efficiently. Fasting is the most efficient form of detoxification, which takes place as the kidneys, lungs, liver, lymph glands, colon, and skin neutralize or dispose of harmful toxins. When you fast, toxins and chemicals that are typically absorbed through your food, skin, and the environment are released. Detoxing is sped up when you fast and your body breaks down fat cells. You may be surprised at the amazing things your body can do, especially since society is told to schedule doctor visits at the slightest sign of illness. As modern medicine has allowed some illnesses and conditions to be cured faster, the medical and pharmaceutical industries have led us to rely on manmade remedies rather than our own bodies to heal us.

As long as you treat your body right and provide it with efficient nutrients, it can still function smoothly. Below is a list of the incredible things that fasting can do for your body...

- Stabilizing Your Leptin Levels. As you already know, leptin is a fat burning hormone that comes in handy when you are trying to lose weight. When you stop consuming a large amount of carbohydrates and sugar on a daily basis, your body becomes for sensitive to leptin, which leads to weight loss.

- Lowers your risk of developing type one and type two diabetes. Some patients have even cured their type two diabetes with fasting and a clean diet.

- Oxidative stress can lead to premature aging and chronic diseases such as: cancer, cardiovascular disease, atherosclerosis, chronic inflammation, myocardial infarction, and more. Multiple studies have shown that fasting improves your body's resistance to oxidative stress.

- Several studies have shown that intermittent fasting helps fight inflammation. Inflammation causes many common conditions and diseases, such as: signs of aging, cancer, diabetes, heart disease, viral and bacterial infections, acid reflux, high blood pressure, urinary tract infections, high blood pressure, and more.

- Heart disease kills more than six hundred thousand people in the United States each year. Intermittent fasting has been proven to decrease the risk of heart disease and other risk factors that are associated with it, such as: high blood pressure, higher LDL cholesterol, high blood sugar levels, and blood triglycerides. Fasting also improves your cardiovascular function by preventing obstructed arterial blood flow.

- Autophagy is the deconstruction of cells in your body, in which your body destroys old, sick cells and replaces them with new ones. When you are in a fasting state, your body beings the process of autophagy. This has been shown to protect people against multiple diseases, including cancer and Alzheimer's.

- Fasting will lower and normalize your blood pressure.

- Fasting will control and regulate your appetite over time. The change in your eating patterns and habits will become normalized, which will reduce your appetite and lead you to eat less during your feasting period.

- Intermittent fasting releases hormones in your body that increase the rate of your metabolism. This means that you will burn more calories as you end your fast and begin eating again.

- Fasting gives your digestive system a rest. Eating three or more meals a day puts a lot of stress on your digestive system, which can lead to irregular bowel movements, gas, an overloaded digestive tract, and change the bacteria in your stomach.

- As your body removes old cells and replaces them with new ones, your body will begin to change. Your skin will be healthier and any acne will go away, damaged organs will heal, and your lifespan will increase.

- Along with being known to prevent and cure cancer, fasting has also been proven to improve the symptoms of chemotherapy and increase the effectiveness of the treatment.

- Fasting will improve neurogenesis and neuronal plasticity, which protects you against and cleanses any neurotoxins and other harmful toxins that can inhibit healthy brain function.

These are just the most effective benefits that fasting can bring. Many fasting participants have found significant changes in their health, from curing type two diabetes to having more energy during the day. But there are other miraculous effects that you will experience after a few weeks of intermittent fasting. These may include:

- A better attitude

- Better sleeping patterns with more REM sleep

- Centralized thoughts and increased focus

- Clearer scheduling and planning

- Increased motivation and energy

- Stronger willpower and self- discipline

- Drug detoxification; if you take prescription medicine or pain killers regularly, you will not need to rely on them as much as you have before.

- Increased creativity and productivity

- Improved senses; such as vision, taste, and hearing.

- Mental, emotional, and spiritual clarity

- A more relaxed mind and body

- Reduced allergies

- Cured or prevented obesity

- More relaxed bowel movements and gas relief

- Rejuvenation and revitalization

Chapter 4: Common Myths of Intermittent Fasting

When it comes to losing weight everyone seems to have their own two cents worth of advice to give. Even you have probably offered someone a tip or two about losing weight at one point or another. Today, information is available at the tips of your fingers. You can look up dozens of different weight loss programs on your phone, tablet, computer, in magazines, and books. Most of the time you can't go a day without turning on the television and seeing a commercial for a new "miraculous" supplement, waist shaper, or exercise DVD.

Surveys have shown that more than fifty percent of women in the United States are on a diet at any given moment. So chances are you have already talked to your girlfriends or relatives about fasting and have received a number of different responses. But the fact of the matter is that there are many myths about fasting and intermittent fasting that have become common knowledge that may make you doubt your decision to make this change. In this chapter I am going to debunk the most well- known myths about intermittent fasting, so you understand the full effects of this lifestyle.

1. Fasting is Basically Starving Yourself

Possibly the greatest myth about fasting is that you are starving your body of food. Starving obviously isn't healthy and is attributed to serious eating disorders. But fasting is not an eating disorder nor is it starvation. In fact, intermittent fasting helps individuals develop stable and regular eating habits. Starvation is when you rob your body of food; you purposely do not give it any source of food, resulting in malnourishment and even death. Fasting is when the participant chooses select times to feed their body the proper nutrients it needs. Not only are you making better choices when you fast, but you are also giving your digestive system a rest. You cannot become seriously injured or die from fasting, because the point of intermittent fasting is that you *do* break the fast with a delicious meal.

2. Fasting Will Slow Down Your Metabolism

Your metabolism is the energy used to keep your cells active and alive, it sustains your life. While it is true that your metabolic rate effects your weight, intermittent fasting will not slow it down. Research has proven time and time again that the quantity of the food you consume matters, not your eating pattern. This means that how often you eat or when you eat does not correlate with your body composition. What really matters is how much food you eat in regards to your body composition and weight. Of course, when it comes to health, quality matters a great deal as well. Your metabolism is not a mystical fire that you should try to speed up. It is something that you should try to optimize. Fasting will not decrease your metabolism or put your body into starvation mode. Your metabolism will burn however many calories it can, and the only way it will burn more calories for energy is if you also exercise. As long as you eat in a caloric deficit and/ or exercise, you will lose weight.

3. You Will Gain Back The Weight You Lost After Eating

Another common myth is that fasting is a waste of your time because you will just gain back whatever weight you lose as soon as you stop fasting. The only way you will gain back whatever fat you lost is if you do not adapt fasting as a lifestyle and continuously eat after you stop fasting regularly. Fasting is a long-term (*permanent*) solution. I understand that your goal with intermittent fasting may be to lose ten or fifteen pounds. But before you began fasting, you knew that you consumed too many calories during the day; that is why you are reading this book. Fasting will reverse your reliance on excess calories. And stopping a fasting lifestyle will in turn reverse your eating habits right back to overeating and consuming excess calories. Intermittent fasting is not a temporary, quick fix solution to losing a few pounds after a few weeks of minimal effort. In that case, you will find yourself right back where you started. The point of fasting then feasting is to plan your meals and make better decisions during your eating period. Weight gain will only occur if you overcompensate during meals by overeating.

4. Fasting Only Helps You Lose Water Weight

As with many diets, it is a common myth that when you lose weight you are actually losing water weight or muscle glycogen. While this does occur for some people, it is not necessarily true. You absolutely will lose weight in the form of body fat when you fast; it just don't be in the first two weeks of intermittent fasting. As long as you stick to your fasting schedule and plan, you will lose that stubborn belly fat.

5. Having Less Energy When Fasting

Some people believe that because you are eating less food when you adopt intermittent fasting, you experience a lack of energy. When you first begin fasting, you may experience a slight decrease in energy. But once your mind and body adapt to the change in lifestyle, you will actually have increased energy levels, even when skipping meals. The first week or so is the hardest, as it is with any other lifestyle change. When you are hungry, that is when you will expend the most energy. You can use hunger as motivation to stay strong in your goals and stay active and focused on other important tasks. If you keep yourself distracted throughout your fasting period, intermittent fasting is a much more pleasant experience.

6. Fat Makes You Fat

Many people choose to adapt much healthier diets when they take on intermittent fasting. One of the most common myths of losing weight through dieting is that eating fat will make you fat. But this is simply not true. Humans cannot live without fats; they are crucial for our survival. But there is a difference between good fats and bad fats. Good fats give us necessary fatty acids and vitamins, energize us, and keep our skin super soft. The combination of bad fats and carbohydrates is what makes people gain weight, not the consumption of fat. There are even studies that have shown a short term high fat, low carb diet will help you lose more weight than other typical dieting methods.

7. Your Brain Will Stop Functioning Without Carbs

Another myth about dieting and intermittent fasting is that if you do not consume carbohydrates every few hours, your brain will stop working. This belief comes from the theory that your brain can only use glucose to convert to energy. But your body can produce its own glucose through a process called gluconeogenesis. And your body has stored glycogen in the liver that can be used for energy. Lastly, long- term fasting or low carb diets will force your body to produce ketone bodies, which will also energize your brain. The fact of the matter is that our bodies are more than capable of surviving without a constant supply of carbohydrates. If this was not the case, humans would have been extinct long ago.

8. You Need Supplements To Make Up for Lack of Food

There are dozens of different supplements that "experts" claim your body needs during a fasting period. But you don't need green tea pills or raspberry ketones to lose weight and stay motivated during your fast. All your body needs is water.

9. Fasting and Training Are a Bad Combination

While some aerobic activities, such as running, may have a slight negative impact on performance, anaerobic performance, like lifting weights is not as effected by intermittent fasting. Although carbohydrates boost your energy while exercising, a key factor to a good workout is staying hydrated. The most common type of athlete that participates in intermittent fasting is a weight trainer or lifter. And luckily for athletes who are focused on changing their body composition, fasting allows your body to lose fat while still gaining muscle: as long as you feast with the right kinds of food.

When Fasting Is Not For Everyone ...

As you now know, fasting can effect women differently than men; which means that there are limitations to who can or should fast and who cannot. There are also a number of other factors that come into play when deciding if you should fast, like stress and eating disorders.

You should not try intermittent fasting if:

- You are pregnant - This is because pregnant women have a higher demand for more energy and nutrients that come from what they eat and drink. But really, some women should not even try experimenting with intermittent fasting at all. If you do not feast or fast properly, you risk become infertile or early onset menopause: even if you are in your twenties.

- You having a history of any kind of eating disorder – Individuals who have suffered from an eating disorder are more likely to develop another eating disorder at some point in their lives. Fasting and feasting could lead patients with unhealthy eating patterns to develop additional problems.

- You are chronically stressed or do not handle physical or mental stress well – people who experience constant chronic stress should not limit their diet or meals because they may actually need more nourishment.

- You have insomnia or unusual sleeping habits – Just like individuals with chronic stress, if you have trouble sleeping, then you need to be nurturing your body not adding more stress.

- If you are new to exercising and dieting and this is the first time you are trying a new lifestyle.

Now that you fully understand the science behind fasting, as well as the many benefits and myths behind the method, you are now prepared to read all about the different types of intermittent fasting plans. Everyone has their own needs when it comes to incorporating a new lifestyle; Jill may work a full time job and have a family to take care of, while Katie is a full time student who works out five days a week. Whatever your needs are, there is a way to adopt intermittent fasting without it disrupting your everyday life. Keep reading onto chapter five to learn more about the most popular fasting methods.

Chapter 5: Popular Fasting Methods and Programs

There are a number of different intermittent fasting methods that can be incorporated by athletes or any woman who just wants to lose a few pounds. This chapters lists and explains the most commonly practices methods, so you can choose a plan that is right for you.

The 16 Hour Fast; The 16:8 Diet

The 16:8 method is very popular and makes intermittent fasting a much more sustainable lifestyle. During a sixteen hour fast, you restrict your feasting period to just eight hours a day, then follow with a sixteen hour fasting period. For example: if your last meal was a six o'clock at night on Tuesday, you would fast until ten o'clock the next morning. This method allows you to continue eating the yummy food you love in two meals a day, and you are allowed to snack too. The key to a sixteen hour fast is making sure that you are fasting when you are sleeping, so you do not experience any cravings. One characteristic of the sixteen hour fast is that you practice is every day.

Eat- Stop- Eat

The eat- stop- eat plan involves fasting for a longer period of time a few days a week. While practicing this method, the participant will fast for a full twenty-four hours once or twice a week. For example: if your last meal on Wednesday was dinner at six, then you will not eat again until six o'clock at night on Thursday. A twenty- four hour fast may sound intimidating, but you do not need to do more than two fasts a week. Your two fasts should never be consecutive days, but spread evenly throughout your week. The eat-stop-eat method can be slightly more challenging for individuals with specific needs or who are sensitive to symptoms: such as low blood sugar or low blood pressure.

The 5:2 Diet

The 5:2 diet has become more mainstream in the last few years because it is adaptable to almost any lifestyle, as it is more of a restrictive diet than a fast. During the 5:2 diet, the participant is allowed to consume a certain number of calories during the fasting days, which results in weight loss. This diet plan requires you to figure out what your daily caloric intake should be, and then lower it into a deficit; this means you subtract five hundred to eight hundred calories from what you would usually eat during the day. So for two days a week, you will eat in a caloric deficit, then eat normally the other five days. But once again, your two fasting days should not be consecutive.

The Warrior Diet

The warrior diet is becoming increasingly popular for athletes who are in training. During this method, the participant will fast for twenty hours every day and only eat one large meal each night. However, the eating habits for this plan are much stricter than other methods because what and when you eat play a role in your training. The theory behind the warrior diet is based on giving your body essential nutrients in sync with circadian rhythms. It is also based on the theory that humans are nocturnal eaters who are biologically programmed to eat at night. With the warrior diet, you are allowed to consume raw fruits and vegetables, fresh squeezed juice, and small servings of protein during your twenty hours of fasting. During the four hour eating period, you must eat a large amount of food to maximize your body's parasympathetic nervous system. It is also important to eat your food groups in a certain order; starting with vegetables, then protein and fat, followed by carbs if you are still hungry.

Alternate Day Fasting

This intermittent fasting method is great for individuals who have a specific goal weight in mind and is very simple to follow. The alternate day fasting plan is when the participant eats one- fifth of their normal calorie intake every other day. So for a women, depending on her weight and age, would consume about four to five hundred calories on a fasting day. Then, on the non-fasting days, you can eat normally. Once you start paying attention to the amount of calories a food product has, it can seem a little impossible to eat only four hundred calories. But a great way to feel full and get your nutrients is drinking meal replacement shakes on your fasting days during the first few weeks of this fasting plan. While this plan can fit into most people's lifestyles without a problem, some athletes may find working out on fasting days to be difficult. This plan is about fast and drastic weight loss; just cutting your calorie intake by twenty to thirty percent can help you lose about two pounds a week.

Chapter 6: Proof that Intermittent Fasting Works

Now you have all of the information you need to know about intermittent fasting right at your fingertips. From the great health benefits to just losing weight and eating right, intermittent fasting is the perfect way to achieve your health and fitness goals. Of course, you may not be a doctor or nutritionist, so trusting in yet another diet may make you suspicious of the real results. Every diet and exercise program promises to change your life and help you become a better and healthier you. But it is hard to tell which program is just a fad or money scheme, and which ones are the real deal. Many studies have examined the effects of intermittent fasting, for humans and animals. And plenty of evidence shows that intermittent fasting *is* the real deal! The best part about the various studies is that experiments have been conducted to prove how great intermittent fasting is for you, as well as how it can hurt your health if done in an unhealthy manner.

- Just recently, Amber Simmons, PhD, published an article on easacademy.org that evaluated multiple intermittent fasting programs and their effects. A note that Simmons highlighted was that while many studies have found weight loss to be a great benefit for normal people who fast, there are hardly any studies that document athletes who have adopted the lifestyle. Throughout her article, Simmons cites many studies and trials of patients who have tried fasting and achieved amazing results.

- In 2015, the University of Florida: College of Medicine conducted a study about how intermittent fasting increases longevity and prevents aging- related diseases. The standpoint of the study was to show that while caloric restriction helped individuals with weight loss, constantly eating in a caloric deficit is not a sustainable long term lifestyle. Instead, the scientists proposed intermittent fasting as a more ideal alternative. They studied the effects of intermittent fasting of twenty-four healthy patients and recorded the peoples' hormones, energy levels, and weight to find out if intermittent fasting works. What the researchers concluded was that intermittent fasting works for health individuals who have no underlying health issues.

- In 2013, the Department of Biotechnology at Guru Nanak Dev University in India completed a study of how intermittent fasting effected female lab rats. Their hypothesis was the nutritional infertility was a common occurrence in places where women do not consume enough food to match their expenditure of energy, resulting in anorexia. The researchers analyzed the effects of several hormones and chemicals of the rats who were on the intermittent fasting diet: including leptin, testosterone, estradiol, kisspeptin, and neuropeptides. The belief was that these chemicals potentially affect a woman's reproduction system and energy balance. Thus, the team was trying to prove that intermittent fasting with dietary restriction negatively affected the rats. It was concluded that the restricted eating patterns of the female rats lead to hormonal imbalance, shrunken ovaries, and nutritional infertility.

- There are literally hundreds of blogs, websites, and video blogs that are independently published by regular people who wanted to try intermittent fasting and found out that is works wonders for them. Just by typing "intermittent fasting blogs" into Google will give you a number of real stories of people who swear intermittent fasting saved their lives.

Just like with the individuals who publish their own blogs, you will never know if intermittent fasting will work for you until you try it yourself! You can read as many books or guides as you like, but no one can tell you how IF will affect your body. But if you are still wary about whether or not you want to try intermittent fasting, do some more research until you know what is best for you.

Conclusion

Thank you again for downloading this book!

I hope this book was able to help you to understand how intermittent fasting works and why so many people are doing it!

The next step is to create a fasting plan and get ready to change your life for the better! The only way to get the results you want is to take action and do what you need to do to achieve your goals. So get out a notebook and pen, make a grocery list and fasting schedule, and make a change!

Finally, if you enjoyed this book, please take the time to share your thoughts and post a review on Amazon. It'd be greatly appreciated!

Thank you and good luck!

Made in the USA
Columbia, SC
23 February 2018